I0830909

POTTY TRAINING FOR BOYS IN 3 DAYS

With a Step-by-Step Continuation Plan

A Parents Guide

Nicole Rose

Copyright © 2020 Nicole Rose

All rights reserved. No part of this publication may be reproduced, stored in or introduced into a retrieval system, or transmitted, in any form, or by any means (electronic, mechanical, photocopying, recording, or otherwise) without the prior written permission of the copyright owner of this book and is illegal and punishable by law.

The author of this book does not dispense medical advice or prescribe the use of any technique as a form of treatment for physical, emotional, or medical problems without the advice of a physician, either directly or indirectly. The intent of the author is only to offer information of a general nature to help you in your quest for emotional, physical, and spiritual well-being. In the event you use any of the information in this book for yourself, the author and the publisher assume no responsibility for your actions.

This book is not intended as a substitute for the medical advice of physicians. The reader should regularly consult a physician in matters relating to his/her health and particularly with respect to any symptoms that may require diagnosis or medical attention.

This book is solely for information and educational purposes and does not constitute medical advice. Please consult a medical or health professional before you begin any exercise, nutrition, or supplementation program or if you have questions about your health.

Download Your Free Gift Now

LEARN TO BUILD CONFIDENCE IN YOUR CHILDREN

As a way of saying "thank you" for your purchase,

I'm going to share with you a

Free Gift that is exclusive to readers of

Potty Training for Boys in 3 Days

It will provide you with the tools and guidance to know how to build up your children!

Click Here to Check it Out

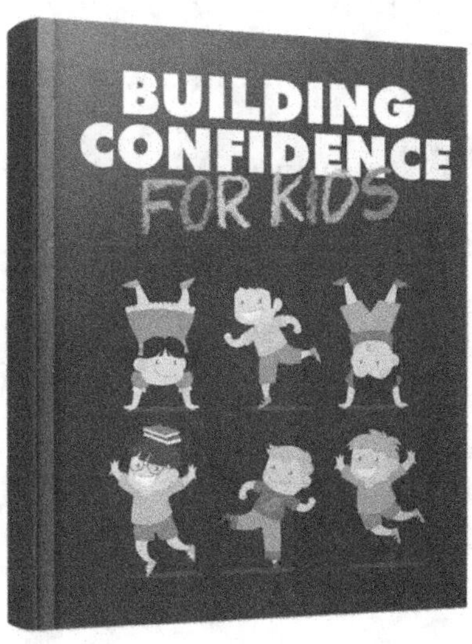

CONTENTS

INTRODUCTION

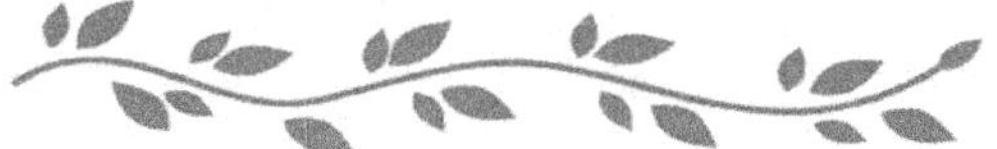

Becoming a parent is the most wonderful thing in the world. Suddenly, your heart overflows with love and, as you are looking at your newborn son, you feel completely at peace with the world. But parenthood is also about challenges, and diaper blowouts are part of the picture. Luckily, there is a time for everything, including potty training.

As a parent, it is only normal to be anxious about getting rid of diapers. Many little boys, however, become quite attached to their nappies and they will prefer constant power struggles rather than giving in to your suggestions. Some children are so difficult to potty train that parents keep delaying the moment and even seek professional advice, fearing something might be wrong with their little ones.

So, what do you do in any difficult situation? That's right. You form a plan. You take action. You find the best way to approach the challenge. Enter the three-day potty training method, who will help your son say goodbye to his diaper in just three days. This is a method that has proven out to be highly successful, and it's time you tried it.

In this book, you will find a guided approach to potty training. Thus, you will support a little boy in his journey toward becoming more independent. Thanks to the multitude of useful information, you will no longer feel anxious or frustrated with your child. The actionable tips will bring you closer to the much-desired dream of seeing your son using the potty or the toilet. They are easy to follow and, as you will read, go beyond the three days for which you will implement the method.

Before you dive in, I would like you to remember only one thing. Potty training should be a fun experience. Support your son throughout this challenge, celebrating each minor success and offering plenty of worthwhile hugs and kisses. Kids grow up fast, and we should enjoy every moment.

I hope you will find this book to be useful. Enjoy your read and, if it will help you potty train your son, recommend it to your friends and family members. Good luck!

CHAPTER 1: THE RIGHT TIME FOR POTTY TRAINING & SIGNS OF READINESS

When is the right time to start potty training? You probably have asked yourself this question countless times. Well, there is no right time, as every family is different, and so is every child. Do not worry though, as children will exhibit signs of readiness, guiding you in the right direction.

Toddlers often go through an independence phase, often associated with the beginning of potty training. This is the phase when they are eager to please, so you will have the best chance of succeeding with this new challenge. I recommend watching for these signs and preparing accordingly.

As the parent of a little boy, it might tempt you to begin potty training at an early age, hoping you will get rid of diapers fast. However, specialists advise waiting until the child shows he/she is ready, otherwise it will take a longer period to succeed. Patience is key, and the best plan for success involves waiting and not rushing your kid into something he is not prepared to handle.

It would also be unrealistic to expect kids to control their bladder and/or bowels until a certain age. For instance, up to the age of 20 months, the pee frequency is high, and it is impossible to ask your kid to "hold it in". Bowel movements develop even later, so parents need to be aware of these milestones before beginning potty training.

Common signs of readiness:

- *Making demands for a wet/dirty diaper to be changed* – the child might use specific words or resort to non-verbal communication, such as grunting; some children pull at the diaper. As your toddler begins to despise dirty diapers, you can take advantage of the opportunity and introduce the potty.

- *Informing about the need to go* – children might say or even shout from their lungs "I need to pee" or "I want to go poo-poo", or communicate their need to go through gestures; others might inform their parents after they went but this is a still a good sign.

- *Understands the words connected related to bodily functions* – whether you prefer using kid-friendly lingo, such as "pee" or "poop", or regular words to describe bodily functions, you have to pay attention and see if your child understands them. The ability to use the same words, in association with the corresponding body parts, is essential.

- *Hiding to pee or poop* – as children become aware of their bodily functions, they prefer hiding. Other children might retreat to a corner.

- *Interest in other's use of the toilet/potty* – some children follow their parents or siblings to the bathroom, trying to copy their behavior. The child might also show specific interest in learning to use the potty, this being connected to his need for independence. Verbal children might ask questions upon seeing a family member, and especially a sibling going to the bathroom.

- *Dry diaper for one or two hours* – a toddler whose diaper is dry for at least one or two hours is ready for the potty; you might notice that you are changing fewer diapers as well.

- *Stays dry for the nap or throughout the night* – a dry diaper for longer than usual is a sign that your child has achieved bladder and/or bowel control.

- *Predictable bowel movements* – if the child has regular bowel movements, you can take advantage of his consistency and begin potty training. It is not important when the child actually poops, it can be in the morning, before bedtime, or after eating.

- *Able to undress himself* – if your little boy can pull down his trousers and/or underwear, he might be able to use the potty with a low risk of accident (especially if there is a sense of urgency).

In beginning potty training, you might also watch for physical signs of readiness. If your little boy can walk without support or even run steadily, you can introduce him to the potty. The same goes for the kids who can sit on the potty for a few minutes or who squat in anticipation of the need to go.

A good idea is to take advantage of the child's desire for independence. Children take pride in even the smallest accomplishment but they need plenty of encouragement to go to the potty. If you have begun the training process based on the signs of readiness your boy has exhibited but the child shows resistance, take a step back and wait. Make sure you attempt potty training during a cooperative phase, and not in an oppositional one when the child says "no" to mostly everything.

It is also worth mentioning that each child develops at its own pace, including when it comes to using the potty. Cognitive development plays an essential role in the success of potty training. You need to make sure that the child understands the physical signals his body sends, whether they refer to peeing or pooping. Children should be able to follow simple instructions and understand the routine associated with bodily functions.

CHAPTER 2: SPECIFICS OF POTTY TRAINING A BOY

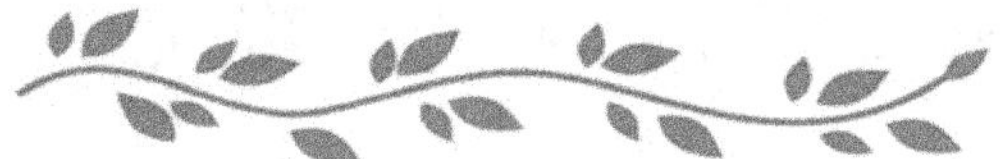

According to child development specialists, boys exhibit readiness skills later than girls. There are several factors involved in the process, including the ability to pull pants and underwear down and back up, as well as a level of concentration and communication. Having a male role model might speed up achievement.

In teaching your son how to use the potty, you will need two things. Time and patience. As for the little one, you have to seek his cooperation and offer plenty of motivation in return. The key to potty training success, regardless of gender, is willingness. Taking the specifics of the gender into account, though, will help you achieve your goals without frustration.

Your son is still a little boy. So, you have to be perseverant and help him understand the connection between the signals the body sends and going to the potty. The potty training process can be scary, so you need to guide him through the steps. Be prepared for accidents but do not give up, as you can become diaper free in just a few days.

Boys reach certain milestones at a later age than girls

Knowing these milestones can save you a lot of frustration and also offer an indication of the right time to start potty training.

- *Age when the child is able to go one entire night without having a bowel movement* – 22 months for girls, 25 months for boys
- *Age when the child can pull pants and underwear down and back* – 29 months for girls, 33 months for boys

Scientists draw attention to the fact that boys and girls develop differently, including when it comes to potty training. It seems that girls learn through fewer repetitions, achieving control earlier than boys.

A male role model to speed up the process

Children learn best through imitation and little boys are no exception from this rule. Dads can show their sons exactly what to do, thus facilitating the learning process. It is said that boys take longer to be potty trained, as the mother is often the one to assume the training process. While it is easy for a little girl to copy her mother, boys might have a hard time understanding the process, as their "equipment" is different.

Sitting or standing?

It is only normal to ask yourself this question, not knowing the right answer. You can begin with sitting, as this will allow your little one to learn that both pee and poop go into the potty. As your son becomes accustomed to using the potty, you can let him decide whether he sits or stands. Remember, the goal is to use the potty.

Compared to girls, boys have it a bit more difficult, in the sense that they have to learn two skills related to potty training. They have to associate the concept of peeing while standing, and to sit with pooping. However, this is only a guideline and you can encourage your son to keep peeing sitting down for as long as he wishes. You can switch to standing up for peeing later. Even when the father models the behavior for the little boy, it can take some time for him to understand the two separate skills to be acquired.

Once your little boy learns to sit down for pooping, you will have another challenge to overcome. Every day, you will have to remind him of the difference between peeing and pooping. Many kids refuse to sit down to poop once they master peeing from the standing up position, which presents a risk of constipation. To avoid such matters, establish a clear routine for going to the potty and keep distractions down to a minimum, at least until your son masters the basics.

What are the other factors leading to delays in potty training?

Here is the scoop. It seems little girls have a higher attention span, being able to concentrate on an activity for a longer period of time. Boys, on the other hand, are more energic and they hop from one activity to the other. So, they might dedicate a few minutes to sitting on the potty, only to jump back up in search of something new to play with. Parents, patience is key.

Communication skills also play an important role in the success of potty training. At the same age, girls might be more developed whereas communication is concerned. As mentioned above, you need to consider your son's level of understanding and also the one of expressing himself before proceeding with potty training.

CHAPTER 3: THE THREE-DAY POTTY TRAINING METHOD

Preparation

First and foremost, you should never begin potty training if your child is not ready. Watch for the afore-mentioned signs and refrain from putting too much pressure on your little boy. Instead, you can actively prepare him for giving up the diaper. Do not rush into this and take a few weeks to properly prepare.

Best time to train

Of course, this is up to each family. Experts recommend though to choose a holiday weekend or even reserve an entire week for the big event. During those days, the child should not go to daycare or kindergarten, as you want to focus exclusively on potty training. Christmas or spring holidays are ideal for that purpose.

The best season to attempt potty training is summer, as being naked is not an issue. Nonetheless, you can give it a try when it's also cold outside, especially since you will most likely spend a lot of time inside the house.

For some children, the underwear delivers a similar experience to wearing a diaper. This is why accidents might be more frequent, compared to the situation in which the child stays naked completely, or at least from the waist down. Moreover, a child who already is naked can be easier place on the toilet.

Free your calendar

Now, once you have decided to say goodbye to diaper days, you need to look at your calendar and schedule the potty training event. Cancel other events, especially on the first day, when you will have plenty of accidents. Outings should be reduced to a minimum or eliminated, as you do not want to take your child anywhere while worrying about him having an accident.

To ensure success, you need to dedicate all of your time to the training process. That might mean giving up on things that are part of the normal routine, including grocery shopping, running errands or playdates. Focus on the potty training, making sure there are no work-related or personal commitments to distract you. You can minimize distractions by asking your partner to handle anything that comes up, where possible.

You can prep some meals ahead and do the laundry, so you won't feel stressed about such important matters. As said, your partner can run errands and go shopping, and you might also consider asking a friend to help you. Don't be afraid to ask, as people are happy to provide their assistance when need be.

Saying goodbye to diapers

Once you have decided to go with this method, you will have to say goodbye to diapers. It is for the best to get rid of these, otherwise, you will be tempted to go back and place your little one in a diaper again.

You can begin talking to your child about giving the diapers away one or two weeks before the actual date. Explain why this is happening and how important it is for big boys to use the toilet. Every day, remind your little one of saying goodbye to diapers, so he is prepared for the major change. When the time comes, place all the diapers in a bag and give them to another family or make a donation.

Becoming familiar with using the toilet

Change is scary for young children. Many kids are afraid of using the toilet, as they believe the plumbing will somehow suck them in. For this reason and many other obvious ones, you need to help your child familiarize himself with using the toilet. Allow him to accompany you to the bathroom, explaining the process and what it entails.

It might also be a good idea to teach him about what happens in the bathroom. You can show them how to flush a toilet, and insist on the importance of washing one's hands. Do your best to make the experience as fun as possible, getting your little one excited about actually using the toilet.

By introducing aspects related to self-care and independence in advance, you will actually facilitate the potty training process. Aside from introducing your toddler to bathroom etiquette, you can also use a doll to model the process.

Mental preparation matters

It sounds good to become free of diapers in just three days. But these will not be easy days to go through. The key is to mentally prepare yourself for what lies ahead, get your head in the right place. Keep in mind that you will spend all that time with your child, so do your best to make the experience comfortable for both of you.

You have a better chance of succeeding by being relaxed. Do not be rigid, as this will only place pressure on yourself and your little boy. Instead, begin with low expectations and be flexible, letting go of any preconceived notions. You cannot be certain everything will go as planned, so it is best to keep an open mind. Just show you are eager, as an enthusiastic behavior will also help your child feel comfortable enough to give up the diaper cold turkey.

Things You Need

To ensure the success of the three-day potty training method, you will need a few things. It is for the best to stock up a few days ahead of starting, so you have everything you will need from the first day.

Potty chair/seat

Experts recommended getting a floor-level potty chair, as it can help small children feel more comfortable with the idea of using the toilet. A potty seat is also a good alternative, and you might try both to see what works.

It is also worth mentioning that a toddler-size potty is less scary. The little one can sit by himself, without fearing that he will fall in. Moreover, given the comfortable position, they can poop easier.

You can decide to place a single potty in the bathroom and teach your son that this is the only one available for both peeing and pooping. Alternatively, you can place a potty in each room of the house, so that you always have one nearby. This can come in handy, especially during the first day, when you will receive short notice about the need to go. Having a potty nearby can save you a lot of energy that would have otherwise gone into cleaning up.

Underwear & socks

During these three days, you will need underwear. Purchase between twenty and thirty pairs, as you will certainly need as many pairs as possible. You can take your little boy to the store and pick out underwear together. For instance, you can choose pairs that have his favorite character, so that he will get all excited about wearing underwear.

For the situation where you might decide to leave your child naked from the waist down, you might consider getting some knee socks. You can also use leg warmers for the same purpose, especially if you have begun potty training during the cold season. If you prefer pants, make sure these are loose-fitting. After all, you do not want to make things harder than they already are.

Fluids & salty snacks

If you encourage the child to drink plenty of fluids, he/she will also use the toilet more often and get plenty of practice in return. So, stock up on water, fruit juice, and water-rich snacks, such as watermelon or popsicles. You can also get some salty snacks, as these will make your little one thirsty. Stick to the regular eating schedule, opting for healthy meals.

Naturally, you want the child to drink as many liquids as possible, to visit the potty frequently and get used to the feeling. However, it is not recommended to force him to drink fluids if he does not want to. The pressure can hinder the process and even cause him to refuse to go to the toilet altogether.

Rewards & treats

You can reward the progress your child has made, using some of his favorite treats or toys. Of course, it is up to you to decide if such incentives are worth using or not. Some parents prefer using non-food rewards, such as stickers.

Supplies for fun activities

As you will have to spend a lot of time cooped inside the house, it might not hurt to think of some fun activities to do and get the supplies you will need. You can teach your son to make pancakes or bake cookies, watch a movie or play various games together. Art projects are also fun, keeping kids entertained for longer periods of time.

Potty training resources

There are plenty of children's books available to introduce your son to potty training. You might also watch a potty movie or use a potty doll to demonstrate the process. Many parents find it useful to try all of these things, including listening to potty songs. What matters is that you get your little one excited about using the toilet.

Cleaning supplies

Accidents will happen, and you need to be prepared. You will need rags, paper towels and towels, as well as cleaning solutions and a bucket. If you have rugs, it might be best to roll them up; a hardwood floor is simpler to clean.

Other

It might not hurt to get some extra sheets and one of those extra-absorbent pads to place under the sheet at night. In terms of food, you might not have a lot of time to cook, so prepping meals the week ahead is a good idea. You can then heat those in the microwave and not have to worry about such matters. Depending on the available time, you can also ask your partner to handle the cooking.

Concern

You have gotten used to the diapers. By now, you are familiar with the process and you have entered a routine that both you and your little one enjoy. However, your son is growing and potty training becomes an important milestone to overcome. It is natural to have concerns regarding this method but, with patience and perseverance, you will see that these only came from the fact you were dealing with the unknown.

Transition to underwear – sudden or gradual?

This is a concern every parent will share. And, like many other things related to your little boy, the decision is up to you. Some parents prefer the sudden and complete transition to underwear after the three days are up, while others decide to wait a couple of months before doing that. In that period, the kids usually go commando, as it is believed the tightness of the underwear can create the false sensation of wearing a diaper and thus increasing the risk of accidents.

Whatever you do, refrain from returning to the diaper. The same goes for training pants, as these are just diapers with a different name. You will need to stay strong and encourage your little one to use the potty. Going commando might seem strange at first but it will ensure the best chance of success. The same goes for leaving the bottom part naked, especially if it is warm outside.

One potty or several?

As mentioned above, this is something that each parent should decide. The important thing is that the potty is accessible within seconds. A toddler is used to peeing or pooping in his diaper, and will rarely pay attention to the process. Nonetheless, as he grows, he will realize what is happening and even be bothered that he is not clean.

It is normal to progress and reach this stage. Keeping the potty close is essential as, despite the realization of bodily functions, little ones cannot hold it for very long. Once the idea has appeared, you need to get him to the potty or accidents will happen. Some parents say that several potties ease the stress associated with the risk of an accident.

Pooping

Pooping is a whole different business from peeing. While little boys might find it fun to practice peeing in the toilet, they can be completely scared of pooping. They are used to the diaper and, now, all of a sudden, we ask them to poop in the potty. As the parent, it is normal to be concerned about this step and fear constipation might become an issue.

Encouragement is all a child needs to overcome his fears. Tell your son it is perfectly fine to let the poop come or fall out. Use phrases like "that's it", "you're doing great" or "I'm proud of you". What matters is that you make pooping less frightening, teaching your son that this is a normal process. Moral support can make all the difference.

If you notice that your little one strains to poop, you might want to pay more attention to his diet. Constipation is often associated with a diet rich in processed foods, bread, bread and dairy. Change the daily meals to include more fresh fruits and vegetables, as well as whole grains.

Accidents

No matter how prepared you might be, accidents are bound to happen. At some point, you will have to clean both pee and poop from the floor. While you cannot always predict these, it can help to have cleaning supplies nearby and handle them as they happen.

When you are done cleaning, talk to your little boy and remind him that both pee and poop go into the potty, and not on the floor. The last thing you want to do is punish your son for such accidents, or make him feel bad for not being able to hold it. Kids are sensitive and they will take to heart what you are saying. The best thing you can do is hide your frustration, avoiding negative reactions or unnecessary punishments.

In the end, it is all a matter of perspective. Accidents can occur and you do not have to become discouraged. On the contrary, change your focus and transform each accident into a learning opportunity. Draw attention to the fact that it is not alright to pee or poop on the floor but do not shout or use physical force to impose yourself.

Keep in mind that little kids do not like change. They like their routine and, when something disrupts it, they are most likely to become agitated. Moreover, being without a diaper is something they did not experience before. Aside from being scared, they might feel uncomfortable. A calm and reassuring parent can help the child process the new stage of his life, and integrate it into the daily routine.

Day 1

The big day has arrived! As soon as your child is awake, remove his diaper and arms yourself with a lot of patience. It might be a good idea for him to spend the first day naked, or at least bare-bottomed. Not only will this increase the chances of your little boy reaching the potty in time, but it will increase awareness regarding the need to go.

Naked is good

A naked child will be more aware of the signals his body sends. You can crank up the heat if need be, letting your little one wear only a shirt and socks to stay warm. What matters is that he can use the potty on the spot, without too much fuss.

Don't forget the fluids

Time to begin giving your little one plenty of fluids. Choose water, milk or diluted juice, as you do not want to load him up on sugar, especially since you will have to spend all of your time inside the house. Once again, the idea is for him to pee frequently, becoming more aware of his bodily functions. A sippy cup can help with the fluid intake, and you will have to be on the constant lookout for signs that he needs to use the toilet.

The basic idea is to offer plenty of practice on the first day, as this will create the foundation for the second day. If your child only pees every couple of hours, it will not be enough to reinforce the need to go. Clearly, you do not want to force too many liquids on him and you should also pay attention to what he drinks. For instance, abundant quantities of apple juice can lead to diarrhea and you do not want to have such issues as well.

Creating a habit

Once you see your son fretting around, do not waste another second. Take him to the potty and celebrate each small achievement. It might also be a good idea to ask him if he needs to go at regular intervals. Some parents prefer setting a timer so that the child associates the ringing with the time to use the potty. After each attempt, teach your son to wash his hands, as it is never too early to begin hygiene education.

If your son has already started to pee, do not worry. Just take him to the potty, as this will help his brain make the connection between a full bladder and the result, meaning peeing. Even if only a drop of pee has reached the potty, this is a small success worth celebrating.

Use the potty doll to reinforce bathroom etiquette, taking your time to show him how it works. Always use the same phrase, for instance, "we pee and poop in the potty", as this will help him remember the basics.

Pee sitting down

Both little boys and girls begin their potty training by sitting down, and this is never an issue. He should first get accustomed to the potty and then practice standing up. You can also teach your son to hold his penis while peeing in the potty.

Handling accidents the right way

During the first day, there will be a lot of accidents and you might find yourself losing your patience. Take a step back and remember that this is a major milestone for your son. Whenever an accident happens, do not lose your temper. Reply in a calm manner and say to him, "we pee and poop in the potty".

Celebrate the progress made

If your child has managed to use the potty several times with success, you have every reason to celebrate. Nonetheless, you have to pay attention to the signals he sends. Some kids take delight in the exuberance of their parents, while others shy away from the attention. Make sure you adapt your response to your child's needs. After all, you know your child best.

Children love pleasing their parents, but they also need to see us glad of their achievements. Make a big deal out of your son using the toilet, if he needs you to do that. You can also offer praise for staying dry.

Use rewards to encourage him

Most children respond well to rewards, so you can resort to giving your child small treats to encourage his progress. Stickers work great, and you can also create a reward chart to use with older kids. Over time, though, it might be for the best to reduce the rewards given for using the potty and instead offer these when your son manages to stay dry for a longer period.

Don't go back to diapers

Sure, it is tempting to go back to diapers, especially if your son is having a hard time using the toilet. Patience. If you want, you can get rid of all the diapers, so as not to be tempted. Some parents, though, prefer keeping a few diapers to use at naptime and bedtime.

Successful or not?

What happens if your little one does not want to go when you ask? Once again, this is a process that requires plenty of patience. Offer encouragement and the possibility to go after a certain activity. Do not pressure your child, otherwise, you will create a vicious circle. The best solution is to get your child used to going at specific moments in the day. For instance, you can encourage him to use the potty before lunch or naptime, or at night, before going to bed. In time, it will become part of his daily routine.

Usually, parents know from the start whether their son will be able to conquer this milestone. In the situation that there are too many accidents and your little one does not pay too much attention to them, perhaps it's best to give him a bit more time. Save yourself the frustration and try again in a month. Never shame your child for not meeting your expectations and, remember, this is a big change and one to be processed in his own time.

Day 2

Usually, on the second day, you will see a glimpse of progress. Most children become more aware of their bodily functions, being able to stay dry for longer periods. By now, you have probably also figured whether your child prefers to use the toilet or the potty.

Repeat day one

Consider the second day as a day for reinforcement. You will have to go throw the same steps, looking for signs of progress. Do your best to get your child to the potty, so he gets plenty of opportunities to practice on this day as well.

Keep offering plenty of fluids to help your son pee frequently and do not forget to plan a day filled with fun activities. Kids get easily bored and they might not like being taken to the potty every half an hour. Distract their attention with something fun to do, and concentrate exclusively on them. Pay attention to the signs he needs to go, as these are still important to monitor.

Short walk possible

Depending on the progress your child has made, you can venture outside for a short walk. It is preferable to do that exactly after he has peed. You can also take a portable potty with you, and a change of clothes in case you venture a bigger distance. Wipes and hand sanitizer should also be in your bag.

The recommendation is to see how the morning goes. If all is well and your son has had few or no accidents, you may go outside for a short walk around the block. You can use each outing as an opportunity to create the habit of him using the potty before leaving the house.

When going out, and clearly depending on the weather, you might give your son a pair of loose pants to wear. Diapers are a clear no, and so are training pants or underwear. Only give him underwear if he's had no accidents during the day and you are sure he can handle the outing. If you are planning on driving somewhere, one of those absorbent pads might protect your car in case of accidents.

Some kids might find it strange to go outside without a diaper or underwear. This is a process in itself, and it takes time for little ones to adapt to change. So, as you are the parent and his number one point of safety, reassure him that everything will be fine. Explain that the risk of accidents is higher in case he insists on wearing underwear or tight pants. Do your best to ensure he feels comfortable.

Accidents are not a thing of the past

Naturally, you can still expect accidents to happen. The rule stays the same. Do not shout at your child or shame him for not being able to hold it in. Always remember this is a gradual process, requiring a lot of patience. Change his clothes when necessary and refrain from making a big deal out of each accident. Refer to the afore-mentioned phrase, "we pee and poop in the potty".

Maintain a positive attitude with regard to accidents. Kids need constancy, including when it comes to your behavior with something "bad" they've done. Explain to your son that anyone can have an accident and encourage him to voice out his need to go.

Naked or not

Some children might exhibit excellent control, so it is normal for the parents to ask themselves whether they should return to undies and pants. Once again, this is something each parent should decide.

It can be a good idea to choose a pair of loose-fitting pants, leaving the underwear in the closet for now. Kids might confuse the underwear with the diaper, inviting accidents to happen. However, if you believe your little one has made real progress, being able to handle both underwear and pants, go for it. Just make sure neither are too tight, so that he can easily get them off.

Fostering independence

Parents are used to doing things for their little ones. Nonetheless, it is important to foster independence from an early age, including when it comes to potty training. On the second day, you might encourage your son to wipe himself. He will show signs of clumsiness but be patient and show him the steps that he needs to follow. Children who are encouraged to be independent often accept the potty or the toilet faster.

By the end of day two, most children have understood the routine and have taken part in the process. Some will also integrate your desire to communicate the need to go, using either words or gestures to express it. Practice makes perfect, so you need to keep going and reinforce the bathroom etiquette.

Even a child who has understood the process might have the occasional slip-up. Children get easily entangled in their own play, leaving peeing or pooping for the last possible second. Be there for your son and offer plenty of reminders, as well as rewards for staying dry. If your child intentionally soils himself, hoping that the diaper will be reinstated, do not give up. With perseverance and patience, you can teach him that the potty is best.

Day 3

You have made it to the third day! These last two days have been intense but both you and your son have learned a lot. On this day, you will have to stick to your routine and reinforce the newly-acquired habits.

Repeat day one and day two

The process will not change. Encourage your child to go to the potty every half an hour, monitoring for any indication that he has to pee or poop. Offer fluids and snacks, and keep the potty within easy reach. Clean up accidents and go on with the planned activities for the day.

Some parents prefer to spend all of the three days inside the house, but that is each parent's decision to make. Practice and reinforce the steps to be followed, and watch for signs of progress.

It might also be a good idea to keep your expectations moderate. Accidents might keep happening, and it would be wrong to assume the occasional slip-ups will not interfere with your daily routine. The solution is to remain calm, change your child and remind him. "We pee and poop in the potty".

Do not force your son to stand up to pee, as there is no rush. Boys can learn to pee while sitting down, but you can encourage them to hold their penis down to avoid accidents, as already mentioned. When he will be older, it will be easier to pee while standing up. Do your best to help him relax and incorporate hand washing as part of the routine.

Out and about

Once again, you do not need to go very far. However, you can stay out for longer, especially if you have a portable potty and a change of clothes. You can take your son to the park, or anywhere else he likes to go, enjoying the fresh air. Going out might also help your son become more confident in his new abilities.

The lesson he needs to learn is that one always goes to the potty before leaving the house. The more you reinforce it, the sooner it will stick. Kids must also be taught that one does not always have access to a toilet. Each outing will come as an opportunity to teach them that they have to control their bladder. So, use the portable potty only when he clearly cannot hold it any longer.

In terms of what to wear, stick to loose pants and avoid underwear. The idea is for the pants to come off easily, without any additional impediments such as undies. Ask your child frequently about the need to go, accepting both verbal and non-verbal responses. Sometimes, kids find it easier to use gestures.

Dry for longer

Some kids can stay dry for several hours at this point, which is great. However, you should keep reminding your little one to go to the potty, to reinforce the habit. Despite the shown confidence, keep in mind that your son is still processing the change. Try talking about the need to use the toilet, and return to the potty movies and books.

It is important to encourage him to speak about the potty and the need to go. Stick to the routine and ask him to go to the potty as soon as he wakes up, as well after meals and before going to bed.

The same goes for going out. Do not ask him if he needs to go but rather make it a requirement.

Time for reflection

While going through the same routine, take a minute and think how far you've come. Celebrate the progress your child has made, big or small. As always, your little one will take delight in your praise.

The first attempt to potty train your little boy may not be successful. If the third day is still filled with accidents and you cannot see any sign of progress, admit defeat. Wait and try again, making sure your child is truly ready for this challenge.

There is a very good chance you will notice a significant improvement in the potty training department. By this point, most toddlers communicate their needs and take interest in their bodily functions. They are also able to make the connection between the signals sent by the body and the potty. So, your effort was all worth it!

Naps vs. Bedtime

Each parent is free to decide whether the diapers will disappear completely at the end of the three days, or if the child will still wear them for naps and during the night. For some parents, it seems easier to concentrate on the daytime. Others prefer to do it all at once, considering the cold-turkey approach to be more effective.

What do the experts say? Some recommend the cold-turkey approach, believing it will be less confusing for the child. Others say that kids require several months to reach night readiness, and this is why parents should only concentrate on daytime training at first. Why does it take longer for night readiness to be reached? It is believed that children need to reach not only a biological age to be ready but also a specific psychological level.

Toddlers first learn to use the potty during the daytime, and the intense three-day process can be quite beneficial for bladder control. Pediatric experts consider that nighttime training takes more time, as control during sleep is a more complex skill to be achieved. Of course, some toddlers might achieve both daytime and nighttime readiness at once, having no problem staying dry throughout the night.

In the beginning, a potty-trained toddler will continue to have accidents during sleep and that is quite normal. This is a learning process and you will have to give him time to reach the point where bladder/bowel control is no longer an issue during sleep. Many parents find this to be the most frustrating part but you have to be patient until the brain makes the connection between waking up at night and going to the potty. As always, some toddlers make this connection quite fast, while others require a bit longer, especially if they are deep sleepers.

Depending on the age of your little one, you might consider involving him in the decision-making process. You can also mention the possibility of wearing underwear during naps, monitoring the child for a few days, noting the frequency of accidents. For nighttime, you can decide whether it is best to wear a diaper or not. By the end of the three days, most parents know if their child is able to stay dry for an entire night.

Each child is different, including in terms of potty training. Some kids will need just a few days to integrate the new skills, staying dry for the nap and even at nighttime. Others might require several weeks to get to the same point. Getting up in the middle of the night will become a common habit, and it will save you from having to clean up any accidents. To reduce the risk of accidents, though, consider taking your son to pee before going to bed.

If you do decide to put a diaper on your child during nighttime, you have to be consistent and remove it as soon as he was woken up. The same goes for pull-ups, making sure that your little one does not pee in them. You can have a talk with your son and explain to him that the diapers or pull-ups are just for sleeping.

Going diaper free for both naps and nighttime will certainly prove to be a challenge but you can overcome it with patience and perseverance. You might want to refrain from giving your son too many liquids before going to bed, to keep the risk of accidents down to a minimum. Make it a habit of putting your little boy on the potty before bed, encouraging him to pee and/or poop.

Potty training can disturb both naps and nighttime, leading to more frequent awakenings. This is a good thing, even though it may cause a lot of frustration. However, when the child wakes up and signals the need to go to the potty, this is a sign of progress. Your son has made the connection between peeing and/or pooping, waking either early in the morning or during the middle of the night to that purpose. Some children will also wake up earlier from their naps because of similar reasons.

If your little one still wears a diaper for naps and/or nighttime, he may wake up because he does not like the uncomfortable sensation of a wet or dirty diaper. You should look at this as another sign of progress, as your child has reached a new level of awareness. Prior to the three-day training, he would most likely have slept without waking up, indifferent to that sensation of discomfort.

CHAPTER 4: HOW TO ENSURE LONG-TERM SUCCESS & ADRESS REGRESS

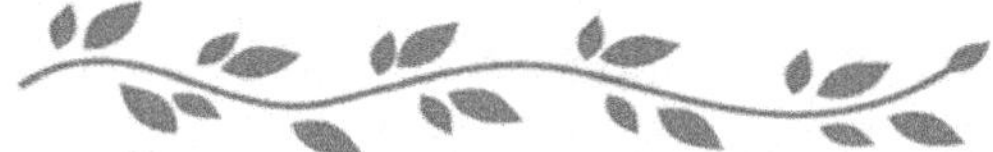

Recommendations for long-term success

The three days are gone and, now, it is only normal to ask yourself: what next? How you ensure the long-term success of this method and get rid of diapers for good? The first thing you need to do is evaluate the result of these three days. If your child has managed to pee or poop in the potty at least ten times, you are on the road to success. You have every reason to expect he will take to the potty in the following months without any issues.

Still naked?

That depends on the child. Some parents prefer leaving the child naked below the waist for another couple of months, still using diapers for naps and nighttime. Others decide to dress their child in loose-fitting pants, with no underwear. Kids who show excellent bladder and/or bowel control may wear underwear but this should never be tight, as it can remind them of the diaper.

A plan for daycare

Naturally, you will have to take your son to daycare. To prevent accidents and eliminate the risk of going back to the diaper, it is recommended to talk to the daycare provider and formulate a plan. Make sure they are consistent, working toward the same goal and reinforcing bathroom etiquette.

It is also recommended to inform not only the daycare providers but also nannies and babysitters of the ways your child communicates the need to go, including gestures and specific words.

Portable potty and a change of clothes

Now that you are daring to return to a normal routine, you also have to be prepared. Aside from putting your son on the potty before going out, you should also keep a portable potty in your car and a clean change of clothes in case of accidents. You might also want to be on the lookout for the closest public bathroom, for the situation that an emergency occurs.

Find the courage to go out, venturing further and further away from your home. In this way, your little one will become more confident in his ability to hold it. When arriving at a destination, take your child to use the potty first and foremost.

Keep practicing

You need to keep practicing until your son masters going to the potty to perfection. The progress will be seen in several different ways. For instance, you will notice that your little one has learned to communicate the need to go, often using a combination of gestures and words. Moreover, the accidents will reduce in number and he will be able to stay dry for longer periods of time.

Wake up at night to prevent accidents

Nighttime accidents are common even in older children but you can keep them at a safe distance by waking up at night and putting your son on the potty. Some kids might wake up by themselves, requiring to go, and this is an encouraging sign that you have done well. Over the next few weeks, he will wet the bed less and less, until you will see that he has managed to stay dry overnight without even waking up.

Keep asking

Just because your child has become accustomed to going to the potty, this does not mean you should stop asking. Why do kids keep having the occasional slip-ups? They might have achieved bladder and/or bowel control but they are easily distracted, forgetting to go until it is too late. The more often you ask, the less reduced the risk of accidents is going to be.

Don't forget it can still be scary

Even if your child goes to the potty, he might still perceive this as a scary and new experience. He might not like the way it feels to be without a diaper. It is your responsibility to stay calm and reassure your little one that everything will be fine.

How to address regresses

There are different reasons for which potty training regression occurs. For instance, when a major life change has taken place, your little boy might want to return to the diapers. More often than not, though, this is only about a power struggle and you need to stand your ground for things to get back to normal. And, believe it or not, a regress can take place with no obvious reason.

Why is my child suddenly refusing to go to the potty?

What do children like the most? To feel in control. Little boys are in a constant power struggle with their parents, and they might choose the potty refusal to make a point. What you need to do is take a step back and give him some space. You might stop reminding him that he needs to go to the potty, making sure that he understands that this is his responsibility.

Some kids might deal with a low level of self-confidence, voicing their concerns out loud. They might say they cannot do it or ask for help, even if they are accustomed to going to the potty. As they fear failure more than anything else, they will prefer to quit ahead. This is the moment to regroup and encourage your little boy to overcome his fear. Gentle and kind.

From as early as they can, children thrive on the attention they receive from their parents. If they may feel neglected, they might wet or soil themselves in the attempt to get you to concentrate exclusively on them. The key is not to show your frustration or shame your son for doing that, but rather offer him the attention he needs throughout the entire day. Try doing fun activities, showing your little one that he is number one.

Emotions are difficult to understand at a toddler age. This is the reason why many toddlers have inexplicable outbursts, as they are trying to find a way to process complex or difficult emotions. During such periods, kids cry more often and they become clingy, and potty training regression might occur. Accidents are frequent when a child is emotionally overwhelmed, so you need to be patient and guide your little one through the process of calming down.

In rare cases, the regression might be just a one-time thing and a poor attempt at getting back at you. Don't worry, as things will get back to normal as soon as you work it out. Take your little one and talk about his feelings, asking him why he is upset. Communication is key.

What do I do?

The most important thing is to be kind. Your little boy is going through a hard time, so you need to be there for him. Patience is key, as this period will pass and things will go back to normal. Resist the temptation of putting him back in diapers and do not give into anger or frustration. It is no use to threaten your son, as this will only make matters worse.

Consequences can help both you and your little boy to get back on track. The first thing to do is to identify the reason behind the regress and impose a consequence for each accident. Attention, each consequence should be enforced with kindness, otherwise, it will only be a punishment and it will fail to serve the intended purpose.

While rewards are useful during the potty training period, they might not be just as much when it comes to regression. Do your best to help your son find his intrinsic motivation, rather than relying on rewards. Asking him to go to the potty just to please you is an equally bad idea, and it will backfire over time.

It is not recommended to make empty threats or say you will take his toys away if the accidents keep occurring. Even a small child will realize that the toys are not connected with his problem but he will understand that you are not treating him fairly. Resentment may follow and that is the last thing you want your child to feel. Use encouraging words instead of praise, and you will what a difference they make.

When an accident happens, ask your child to clean himself and take the soiled clothes to the laundry basket. Depending on the age and independence level, you might require that he changes into clean ones. The enforced consequence should always be age-appropriate and in connection to an accident that just happened. Respect your child and avoid punishments, making sure that each accident is perceived as a learning opportunity.

CHAPTER 5: ANSWERS TO COMMON QUESTIONS

What happens at daycare?

Taking your toddler to daycare might seem scary at first, and it is only normal to be worried about potential accidents. This is the reason why you need to have a talk with the daycare provider and explain everything. Don't be anxious, as they are dealing with recently potty-trained kids on an everyday basis.

What matters is that the child can easily access the bathroom when needed. Some daycares allow you to bring a potty to facilitate the process. It is also important to mention if your kid will require diapers at naptime. When picking him up, inquire whether he has woken up dry from his nap, as this will be a sign things are going in the right direction.

The daycare teachers know how to handle accidents, and understand your little one is still learning. Just pack an extra set of clean clothes and inquire whether going commando is an issue. If it is, then give your child underwear.

Before going to daycare, remind your son that pee and poop go in the potty. Offer words of encouragement and tell him to let his daycare teacher know when he needs to go. If he's had an accident, don't make a big deal when you pick him up. In time, these will become less and less frequent, until they will become a thing of the past.

Can we travel with a newly-trained toddler?

Yes, you can. You will just need to be prepared, so you can avoid accidents. The first thing to do is have your son go to the potty before you leave and again when you arrive at the destination. Never ask him if he has to go, as you are guaranteed to receive a negative answer. Tell him he has to go so you can leave the house.

The travel potty is the number one thing to have for each travel. Not only is this lightweight and foldable, but it can save you the trouble of having to stop and search for a restroom. Kids find such potties to be comfortable and, whereas hygiene is concerned, you can purchase a set of disposable liners. For children who are accustomed to using the toilet, make sure to stop every chance you get.

Pack an extra set of clothes just in case. Choose accommodations where you can wash dirty clothes or research clothing stores beforehand. Pack a separate bag with wipes and nappy bags to facilitate the cleaning up process. It might also be a good idea to get a spare set of clothes for you as well, and seat protectors for the car.

How about using a public restroom?

Using a public restroom should not be a scary experience, but there will be a few things to keep in mind. For instance, you do not want to look for change in your pockets while your kid is screaming that he needs to go right at that very moment. So, always have some spare change within easy reach for such situations.

Do not put your trust in your toddler's ability to hold it. It is for the best to prevent accidents, so stop every time you come across a public restroom. This is particularly important when it comes to traveling. After all, you cannot know how far the next one is going to be and you certainly do not want to carry the travel potty around town.

Of course, hygiene is always an issue with public restrooms. Disposable liners can save you worry, and you will also need hand sanitizer to get rid of germs. If there is a queue for the respective restroom, do not wait. Just ask people to let you use it first, explaining the obvious urgency. It can also happen that your son cannot go on the spot, so do your best to encourage him and do not let yourself be pressured by other people. A simple phrase like "you are doing a great job" can go a long way.

Is going to the pool/beach out of the question?

Yes. But, like with anything else, you will need a plan. Let your son in on the plan, and you will see less resistance. No matter if you are going to the pool or at the beach, take a travel potty and make it clear that he should pee or poop in the potty. It is recommended to use only a few words, making sure the instructions are as clear as possible. For toddlers, it can be difficult to follow directions, especially if you are using too many words.

Remind your son to go to the potty, avoiding any words that might trigger a refusal. You can let him decide on the spot for the travel potty, reminding him that neither pee nor poop belongs in the water. If you are son prefers using the toilet, make sure to identify this first. Show your son how far it is and how long it will take to reach it in case he needs to go. Mention potential issues, such as having to walk on sand.

Swim diapers can be useful. However, you should refrain from using this term, as your toddler might get the wrong idea. You can call them swim pants instead, making it clear that these are to be worn only at the pool or beach. Return to pee and poop belongs in the potty, and reinforce the phrase frequently.

How I handle him playing outside?

It can be tricky to handle playing outside at first. Your toddler has just learned to hold it in, so accidents can happen. Instead of waiting for the worst to happen, it is smart to be prepared. Before going outside to play, have your son use the toilet. You can also take a travel potty with you just in case.

A good trick is to have your child using the potty in different rooms so that he gets accustomed to various physical environments. If possible, do not give your child too many liquids before leaving the house. Take a clean change of clothes and do not make a big deal if an accident happens. Help your son clean up and offer words of encouragement. Everything takes time, including going to the potty outside the familiar house environment.

CONCLUSION

Potty training does not have to be a gruesome experience. As you have seen in this book, there are clear measures that you can take and facilitate the process. Hopefully, throughout the three days, your son will become more aware of his bodily functions and take to the potty as intended. Arm yourself with patience and refrain from putting him back into diapers.

I hope that you have enjoyed the detailed information on the three-day potty training method, along with the practical advice on what should happen next. Before starting the actual training, monitor your son for a few days, and try to identify potential signs of readiness. Prepare yourself for the three days, gathering the things you will need. Remember, mental preparation is also a must, especially since your son might not be so inclined to accept the potty from the first minute.

It is highly likely that everyone will have an opinion about potty training. Listen politely but do what you think to be best for your son. This is a proven method and, thus, it is guaranteed to provide you with the intended results. Accidents should not make you think that you are failing. On the contrary, you should use each accident to reinforce the bathroom etiquette and remind your son that "pee and poop go in the potty".

At the end of these three days, you will still have a lot of work to do. Many kids require time to stay dry for naps and bedtime, so you might want to think about potential accidents and preventative measures to take. Others might regress but, hopefully, the advice included in this book will help you stay on top of that as well.

No doubt, challenges will appear and you have everything you need here to overcome some of the most important ones. Going to daycare, traveling, using a public restroom, going to the pool/beach, or playing outside – everything has been discussed, and I've included plenty of tips on how to handle difficult situations. Whenever you feel conflicted, just go back to that section and give it another read.

That's it. Before I leave you, there is one last thing I want to share with you. Do you realize how big of a step your son has taken? You should be proud of him and how amazing he has been!

www.ingramcontent.com/pod-product-compliance
Lightning Source LLC
Chambersburg PA
CBHW061531250726
48657CB00005B/2175